Things Every Kid Should Know

HAND WASHING

ARSALON NURI

Copyright © 2011 by Arsalon Nuri

All rights reserved.
Eman Publishing.

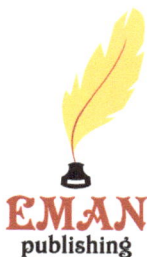

EMAN
publishing

Eman Publishing
P.O. Box 404
FISHERS, IN 46038
www.emanpublishing.com

Order Online: www.arsalonnuri.com

ISBN 13: 978-1-935948-15-5
LCCN: 2011927658

Cover Design by Saqib Shaikh
Printed in the United States of America

Things Every Kid Should Know

HAND WASHING

ARSALON NURI

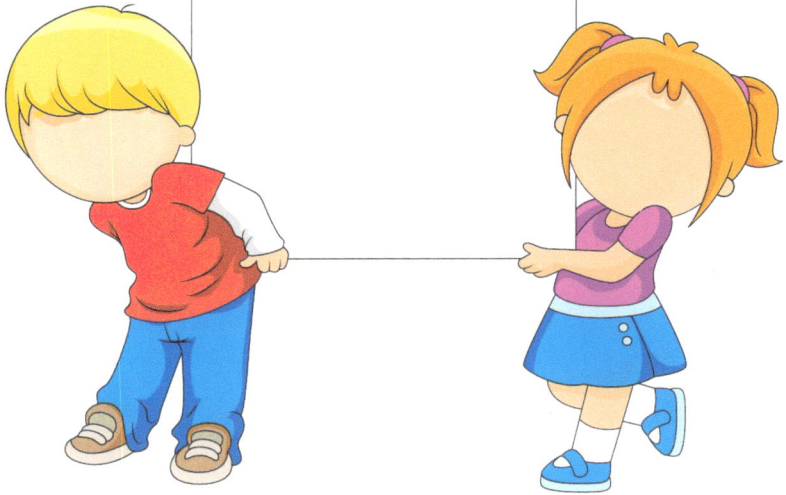

Dan is Kara's brother.

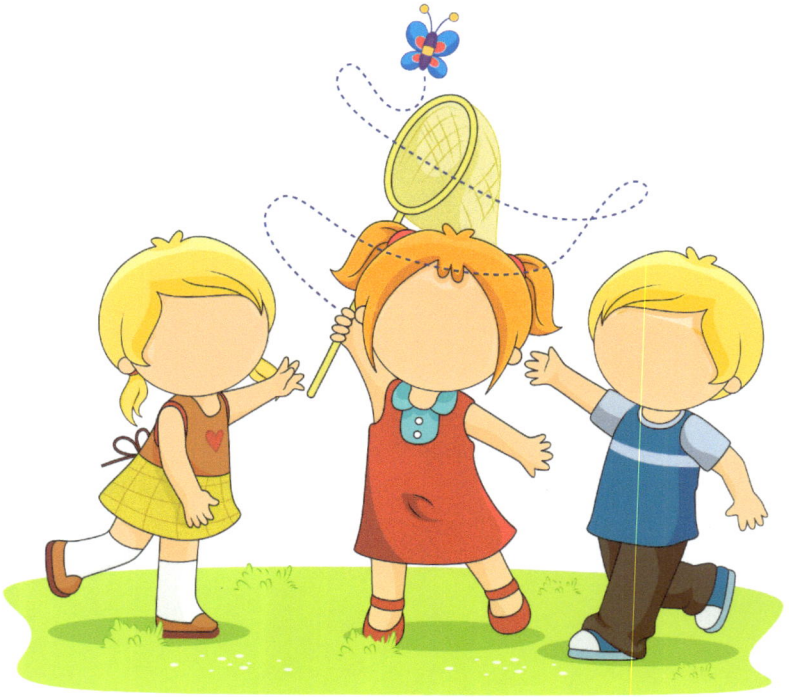

Dan and Kara went to the park.

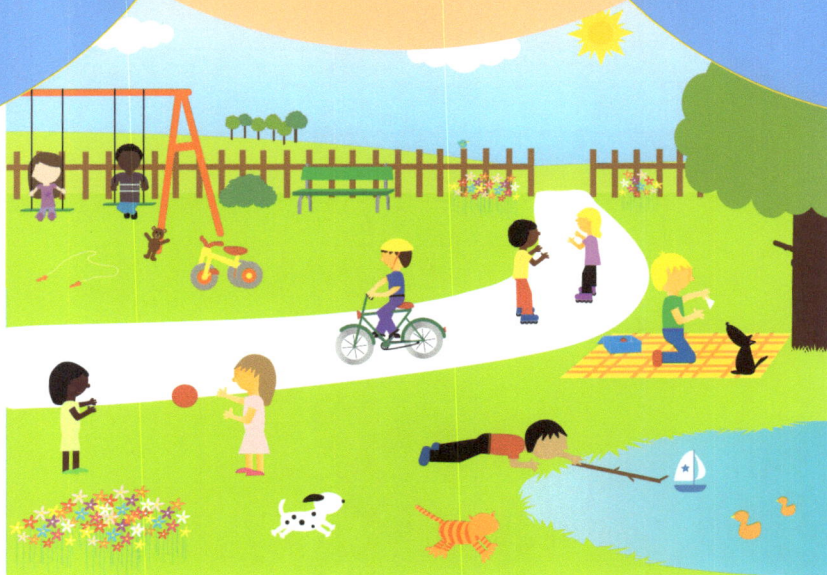

At the park there were many dogs and a couple of cats.

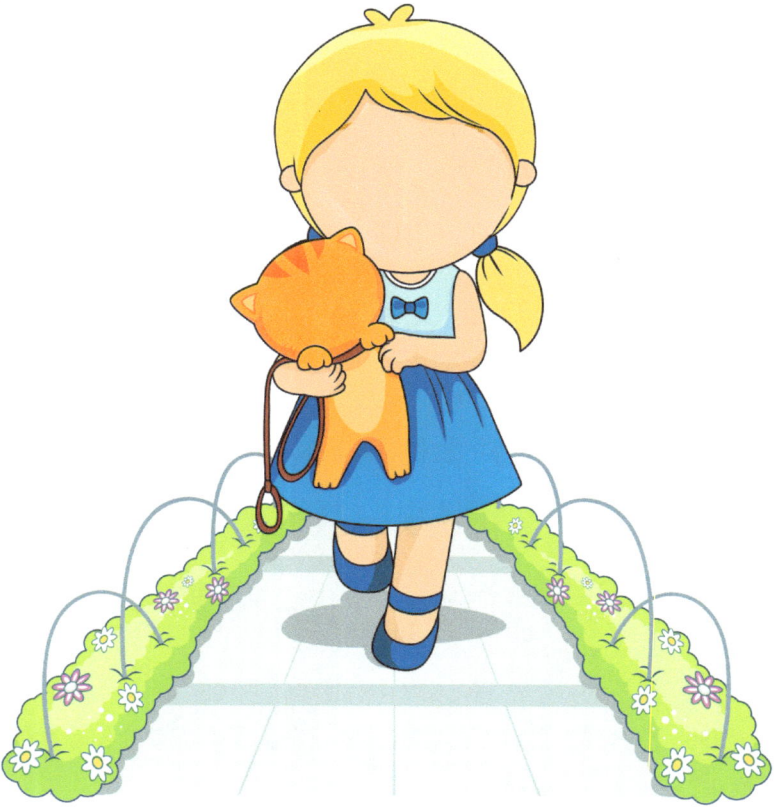

Kara and Dan played with a friends cat.

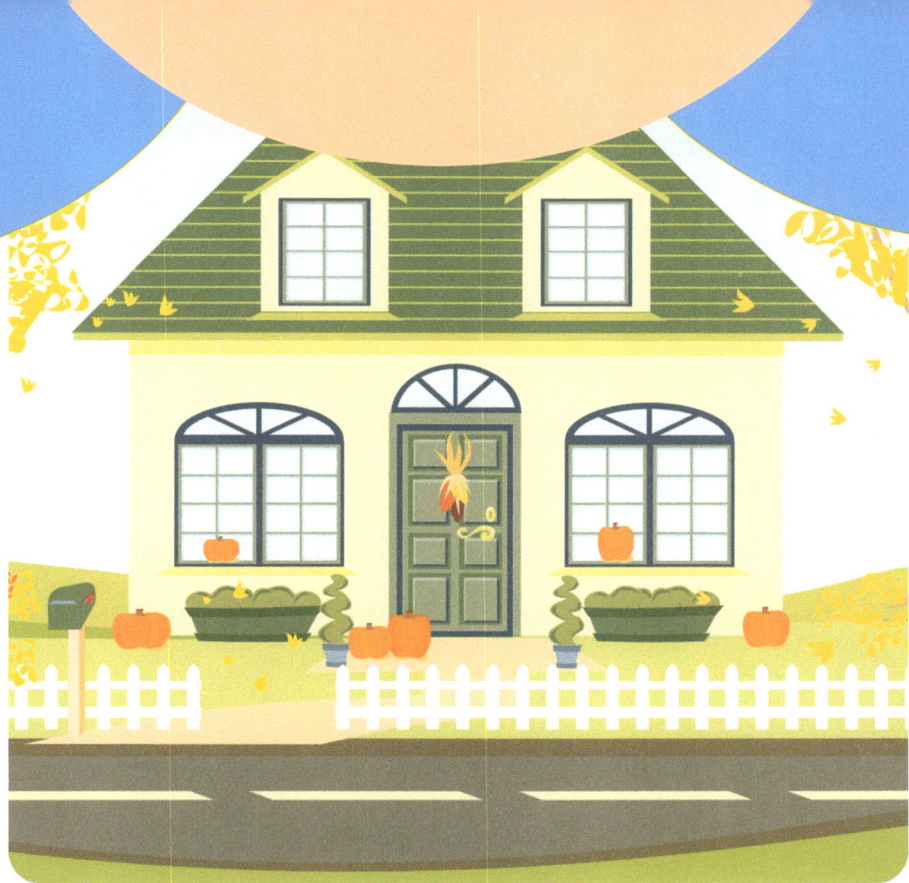

Then it was time to go home.

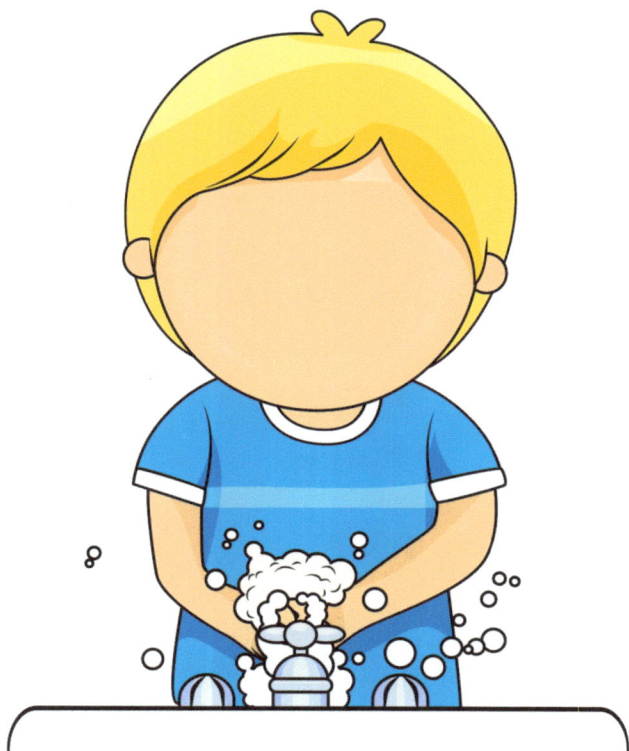

When they got home, Dan ran to the bathroom to wash his hands, while Kara didn't.

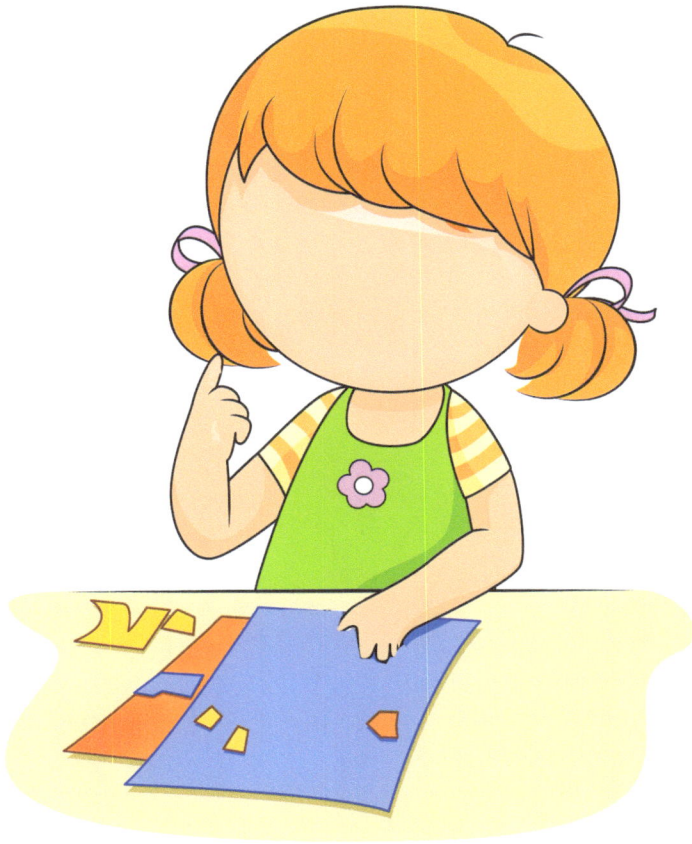

After Dan was done washing his hands,
he asked Kara if she washed her hands.
Kara said, "No."

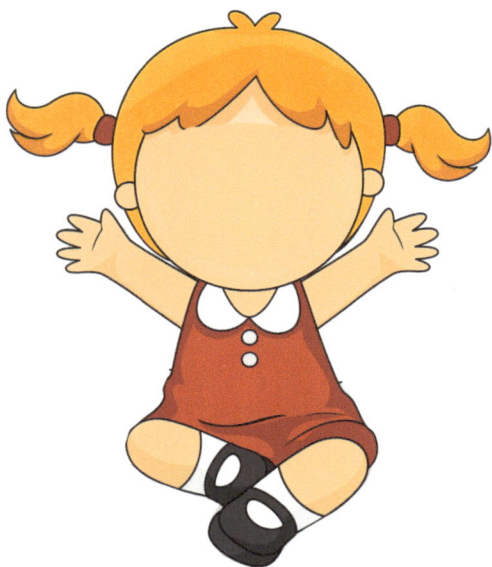

Dan decided to teach Kara how to wash her hands. Kara was happy to learn how to wash her hands with Dan.

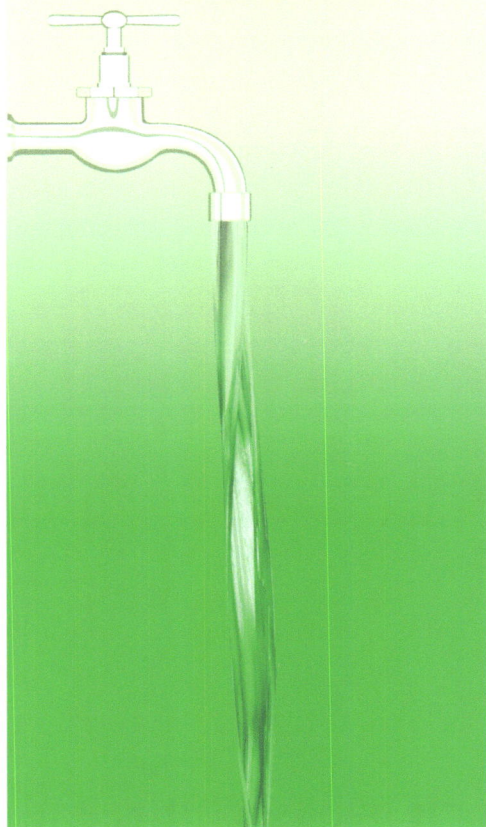

First Dan showed her how to make the water warm.

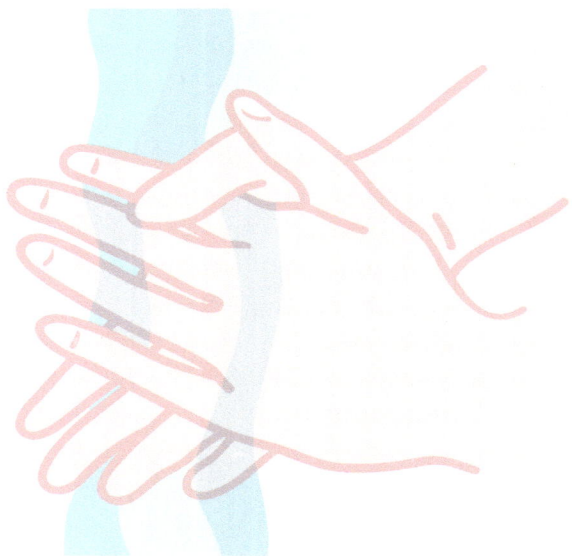

Then he wet his hands a little, and he told Kara to do the same.

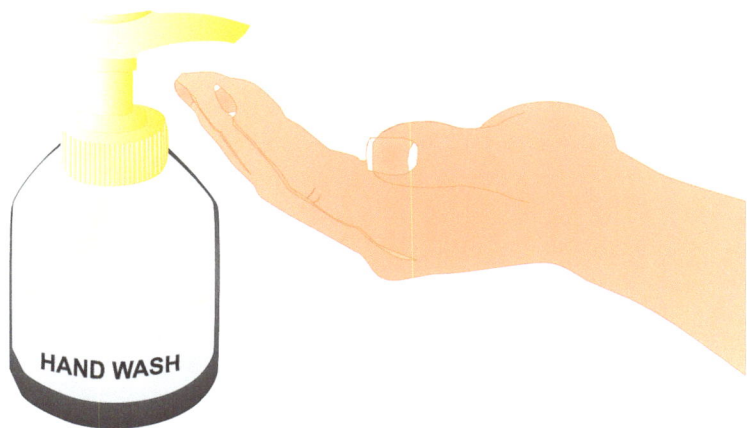

Then Dan put soap on his right palm and told Kara to do the same.

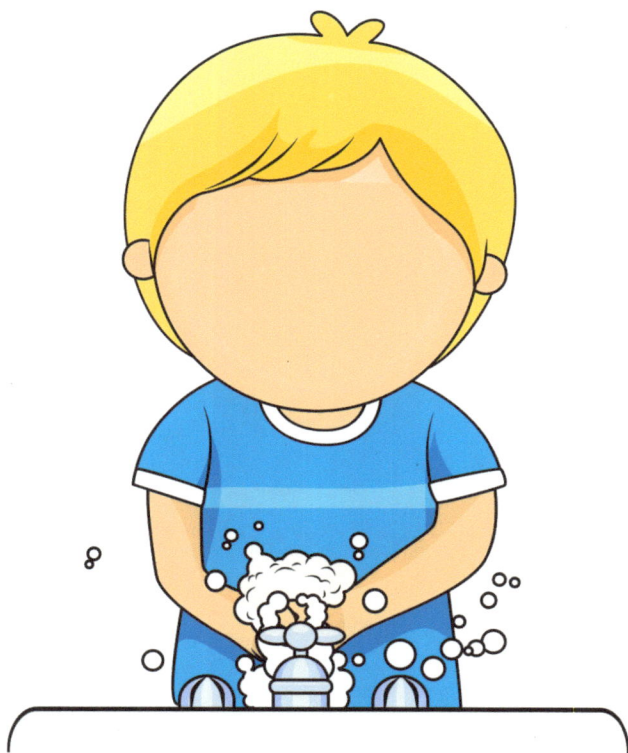

Dan scrubbed his hands while counting to 15, and told Kara to do the same.

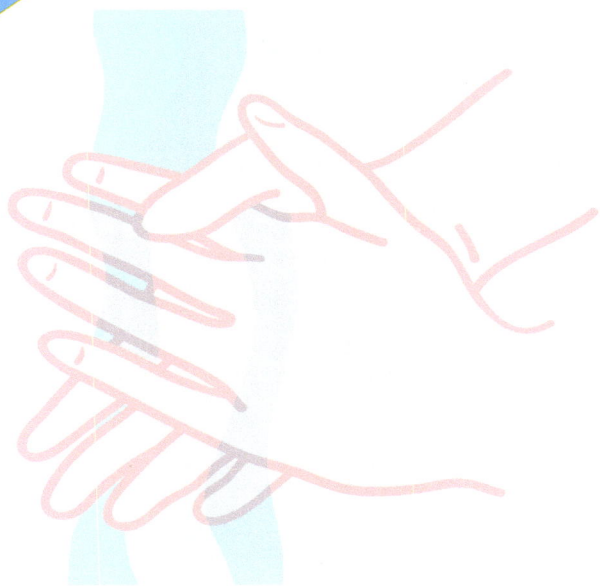

Then Dan rinsed his hands with warm water, and he told Kara to do the same.

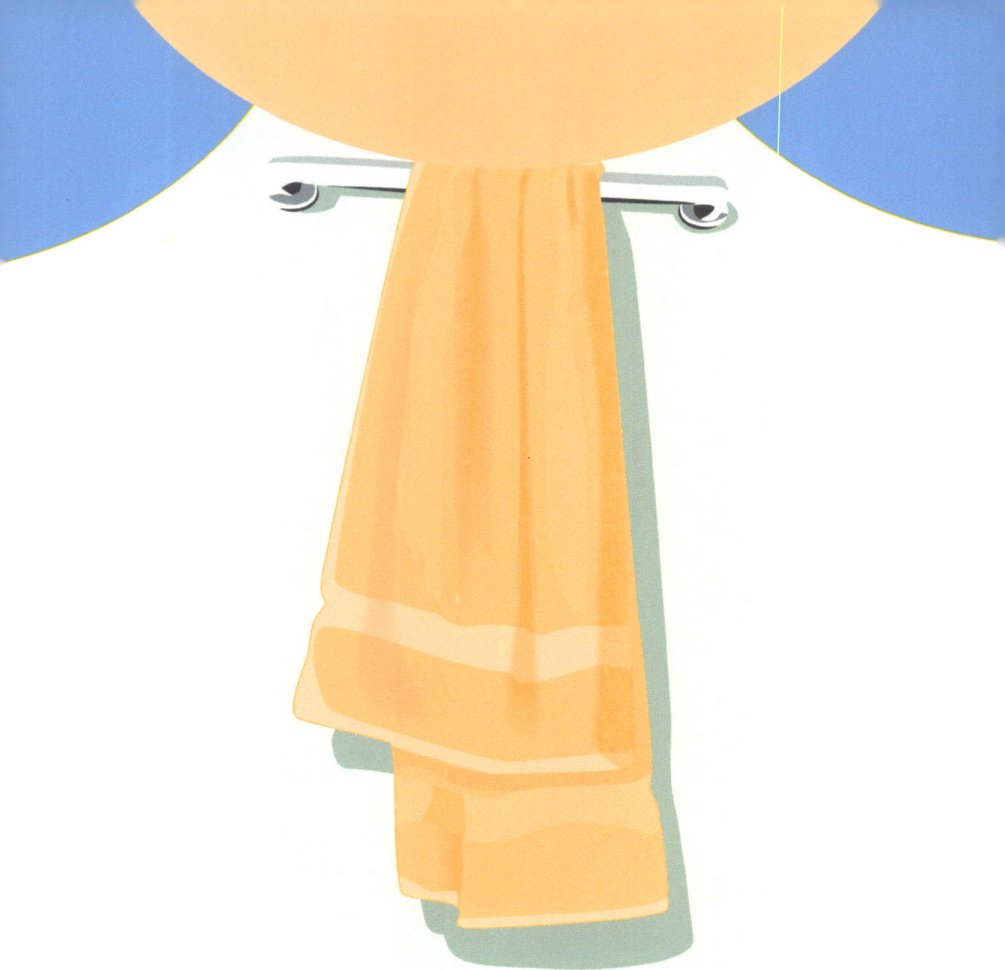

Finally Dan turned off the tap, and he and Kara dried their hands with a towel.

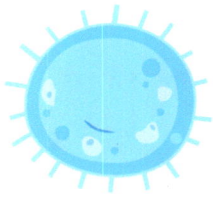

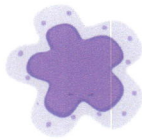

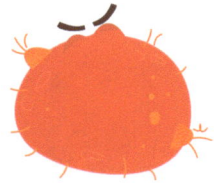

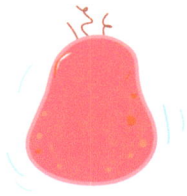

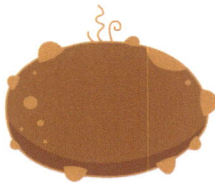

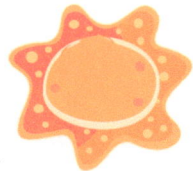

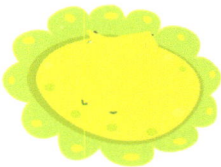

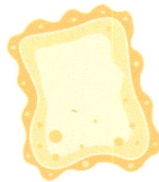

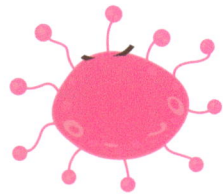

Hand washing is very important, so that germs cannot go from your hands into your mouth or other body parts. If germs go into your mouth or other body parts you can get sick.

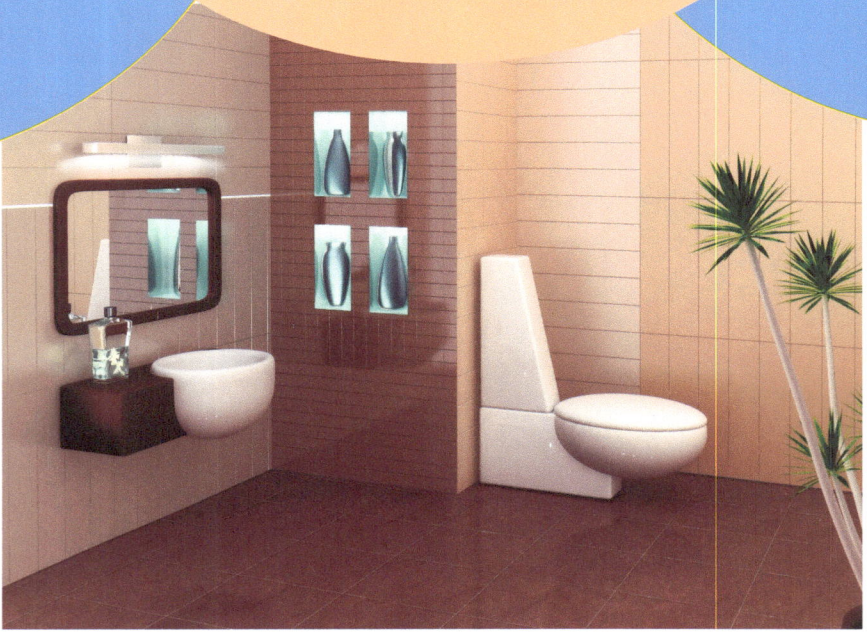

Wash your hands every time you:

1. Use the bathroom.

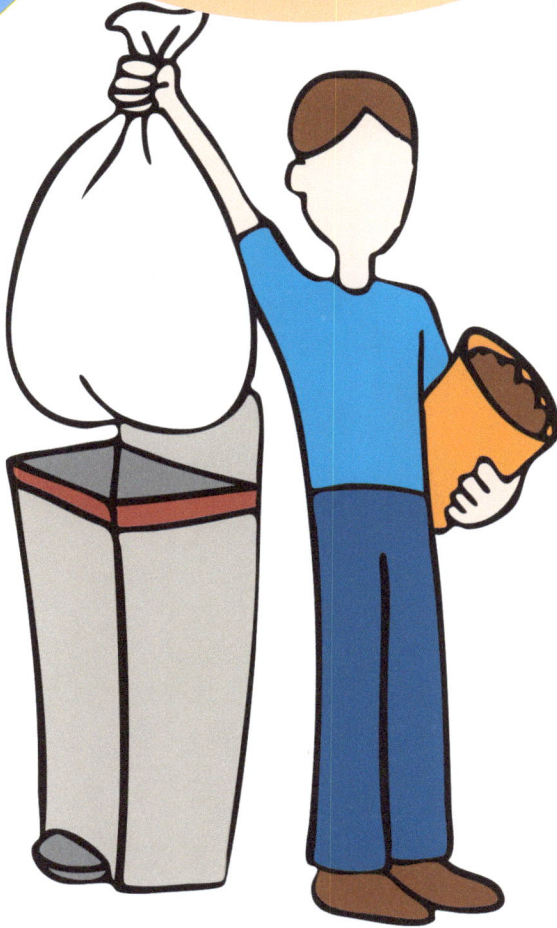

2.   Take out the garbage.

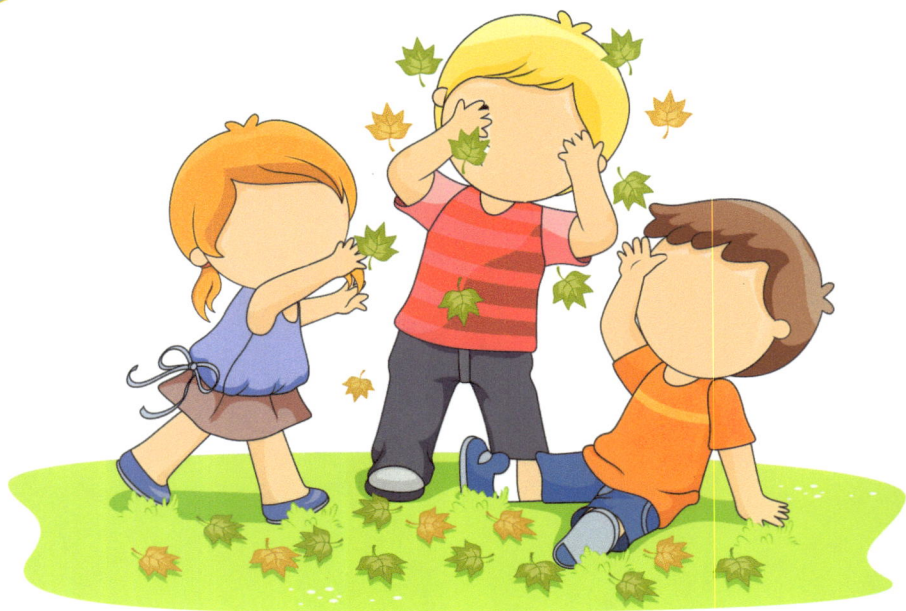

3. **Come from outside.**

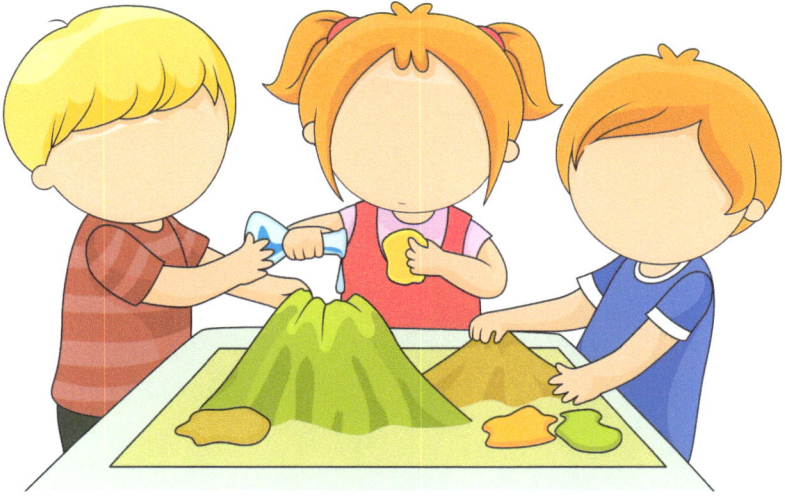

4. **Touch dirty things.**

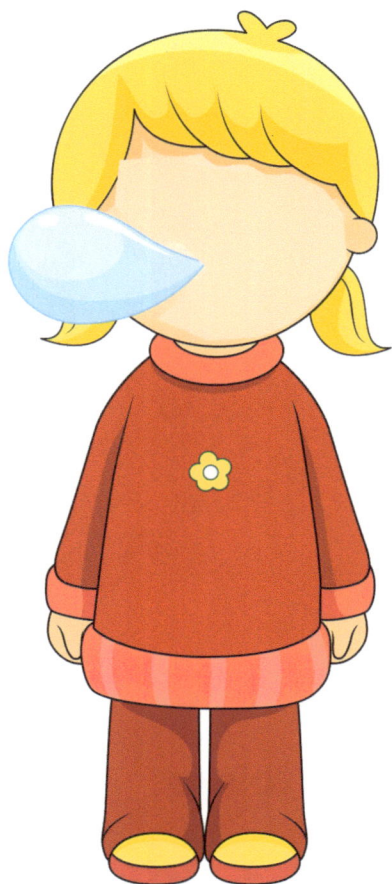

5. **Blow your nose.**

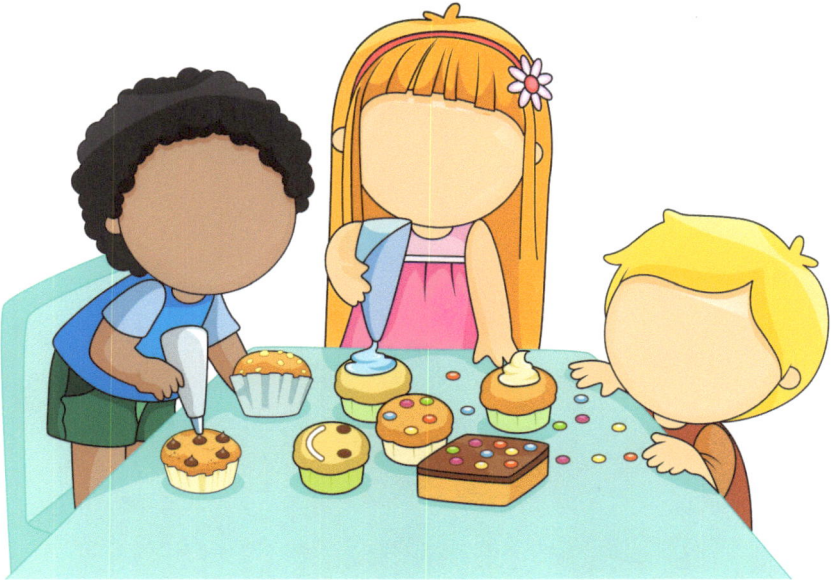

6.   **Eat or touch food.**

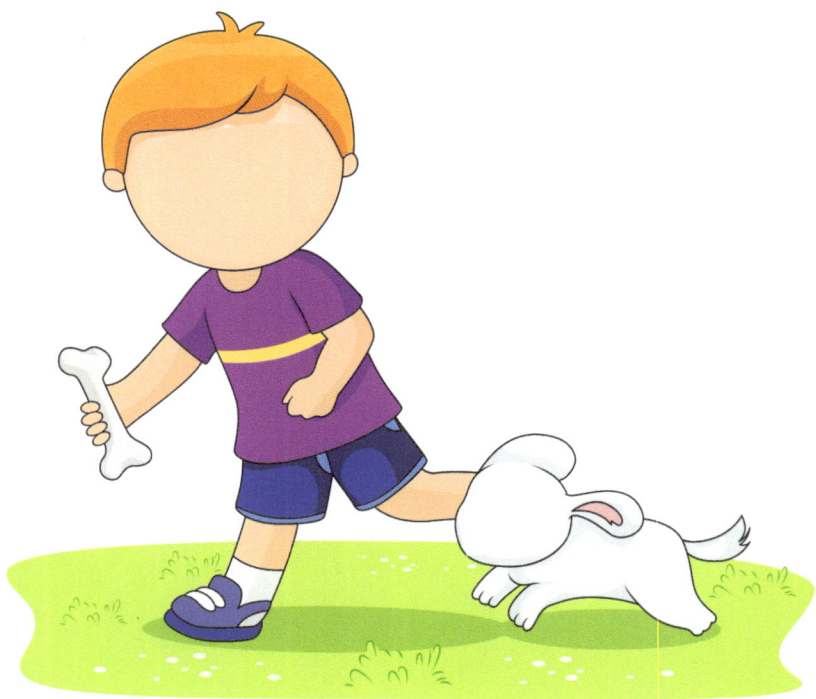

7. **Touch an animal.**

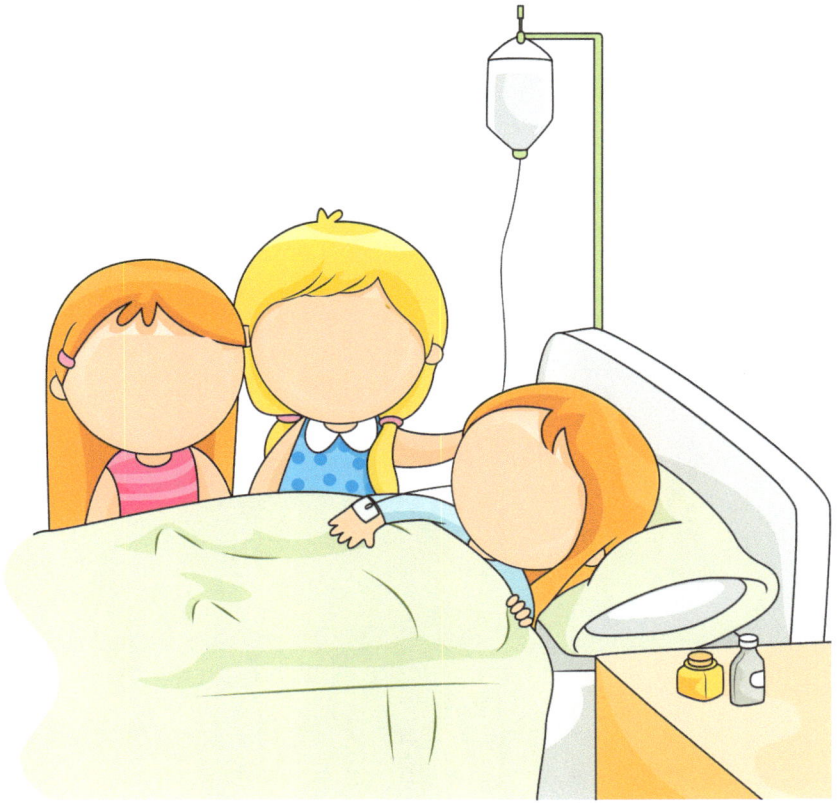

8.   Visit a sick person.

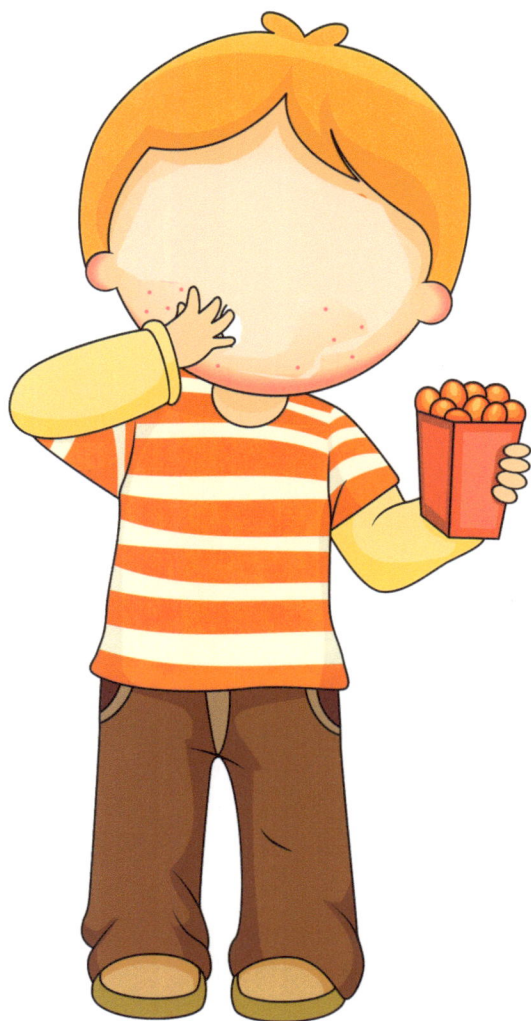

9.   Cough.

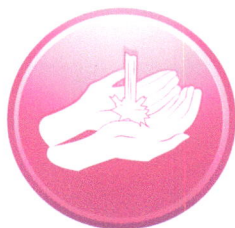

Wet

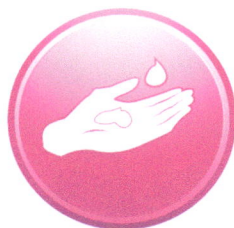

Soap

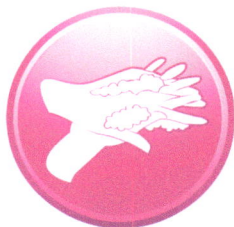

Wash

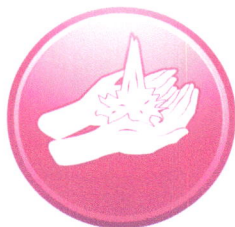

Rince

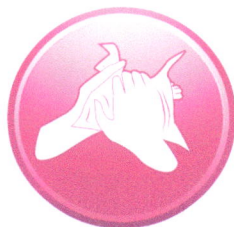

Dry

5 easy steps to washing hands:

1. You wet your hands a little.
2. Put soap in your right palm.
3. Scrub your hands and count to 15 slowly.
4. Rinse your hands with water.
5. Dry your hands with a towel.

www.ingramcontent.com/pod-product-compliance
Lightning Source LLC
Chambersburg PA
CBHW041224270326
41933CB00001B/39